Ring Fit Adventure Owner's Manual

Beginners Guide to Help You Master Your Fitness Exercises Goal Ring Fit Adventure

Gladys E. Omo

Table of Contents

Introduction 1

CHAPTER ONE: UNDERSTANDING YOUR RING FIT ADVENTURE 2

CHAPTER 2: HOW TO GET STARTED PLAYING RING FIT ADVENTURE ON NINTENTO SWITCH 6

CHAPTER 4: GETTING STARTED.. 20

CHAPTER 5: FREQUENTLY ASKED QUESTIONS..................... 26

CONCLUSION... 31

Introduction

If you have made up your mind to stick to the fitness goals that you have set for yourself, the ultimate RPG which is easily accessible has provided enough exercises for you to use as workouts. These work outs focuses on making exercise fun for you. There would be no reason for you to stop, when you are enjoying yourself.

This guide has been put together to introduce you to the basic things you need to know about the Ring Fit Adventure fitness exercise game, I hope you find it useful. The RPG game can be quite easy to start, but difficult to get used to. However, keep it in mind that, this could be your first step on a journey to enjoying better health.

CHAPTER ONE:

UNDERSTANDING YOUR RING

FIT ADVENTURE

Ring Fit Adventure is a game of exercise, known as an RPG game. It was developed and published by Nintendo for the Nintendo Switch. There are two components that come along with this game.

The first one is a Leg Strap, a piece of fabric that you can attach to your thigh, to keep track of your walking and jumping activities. The second component is a circular exercising Ring Controller (Ring Con), a flexible, hard-plastic ring that the user holds, which helps to track the arms and other body movements.

If you want to operate this, you will need two Joy Con controllers. The Joy Con controllers normally come with the Nintendo Switch. One of the Joy Con controllers will slip into the leg strap while the other one will fit into the circular controller.

Once they have been inserted, start up the game, and the both of them will synch normally. Take Note that for you to be able to operate the game, you need the both of these special controllers and the Joy Con. See picture below

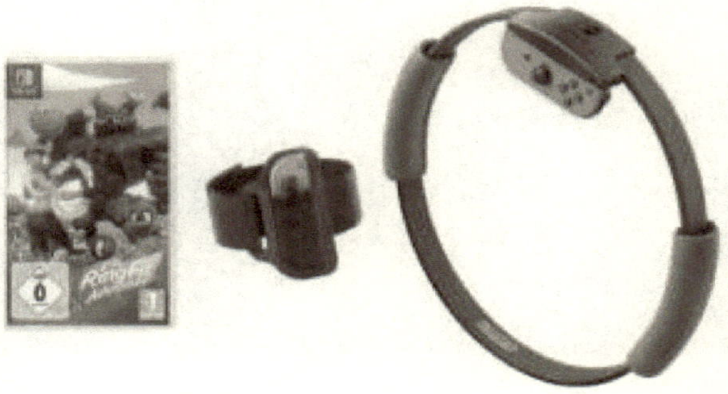

The game has two major modes. The main mode of the game, requires that the player should complete a turn based role-playing

game. That means the movement of the player and his battle actions are based on working out some specific physical activities. And these physical activities will require him to use the Ring-Con and also the Leg strap alongside the motion controls which is inserted within the Joy-Con to check the movement of the player.

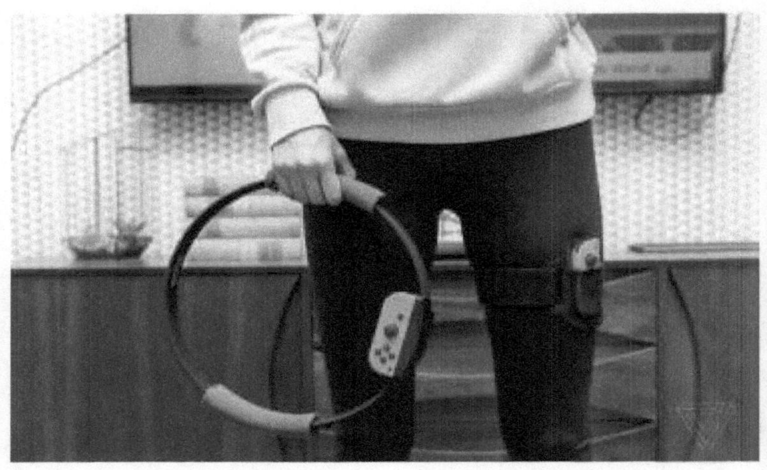

The other mode involves general guided fitness routines and games that are of party style. These physical activities focus on common fitness exercises, and that is why the game is part of "Nintendo's quality of life" goals alongside a similar game of theirs known as, Will Fit. The Ring Fit Adventure game was released worldwide in 2019.

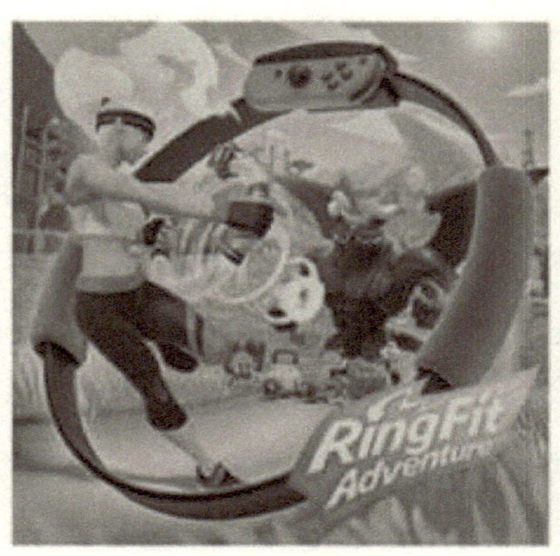

CHAPTER 2: HOW TO GET STARTED PLAYING RING FIT ADVENTURE ON NINTENTO SWITCH

The Ring Fit Adventure game joins Nintendo switch, by making available a new and creative way to get back in shape while fighting with monsters in a fantasy-themed world. It's a wonderful idea and it is one that will benefit you as you get used to the game. Ring Fit Adventure has a lot of mini-games too, these games mixes up with physical exercises that you will carry out using the peripherals that come along with the game. Performing these activities will make you sweat, but in the end it is actually worth the sweat compared to the normal exercises that you do.

In the battles available in the game, you can choose different types of exercises to do in order to fight enemies, because some enemies are weak against certain types of exercises. There are like 30 different types of attacks you can use, and the accuracy with which you use to complete each exercise is what will determine the level of damage it does.

You can also defend yourself against the enemy attacks by holding and pressing the Ring- Con controller into your abdomen (see picture below).

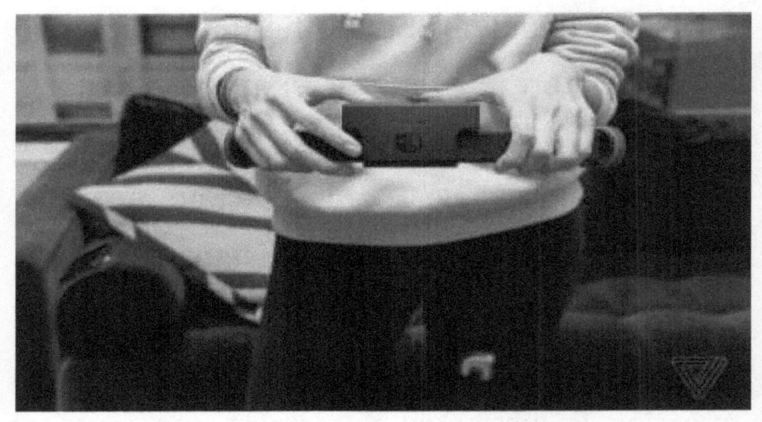

TAKE ON ADVENTURE MODE, OR TRY QUICK PLAY

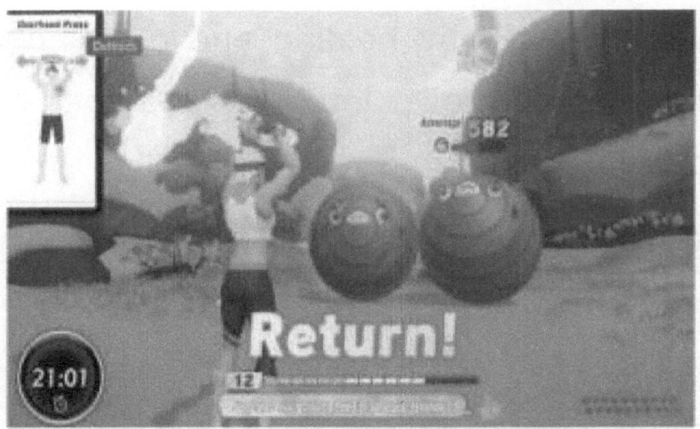

Once you have adjusted your controllers you are now set to go. The next thing to do is to start up the game.

Once you start, you have different options available to choose from. One of the major modes of the game is "Adventure Mode", it is actually the main attraction of the game. From here you will run through the world, trying and making efforts to defeat a supper muscular dragon called Dragauex.

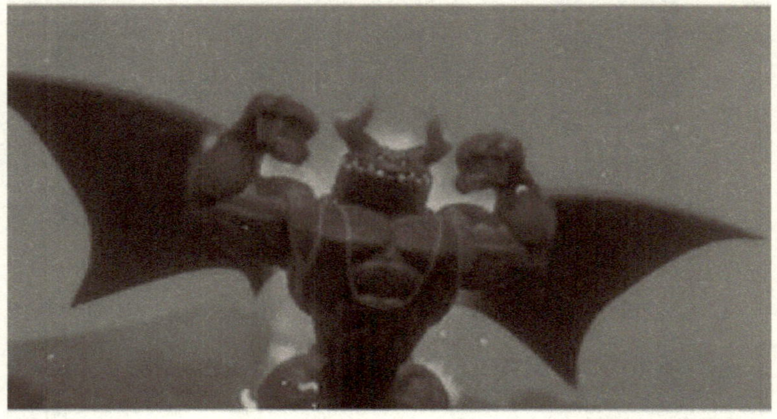

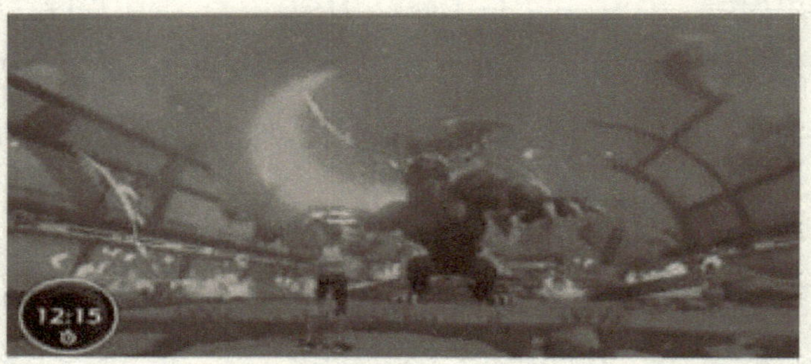

As you go along the way, you will fight with many of the Dragon's miscreants, by carrying out some specific exercises to take them down.

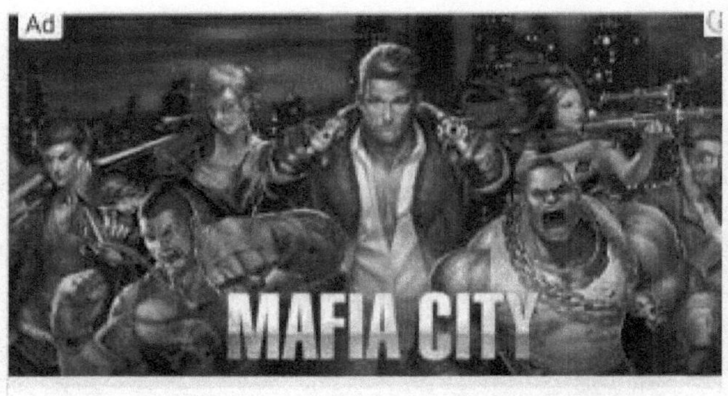

In case you don't feel like playing the complete game, there is a Quick Play Mode that you can play. From the Quick Play Mode, you can play from a variety of unlocked mini-games. Then there are also some exercises set apart for specific parts of the body.

The game has a variety of exercises in all, which are directed towards the arms, chest and legs. YOGA poses is also an option for you, (that is if you are flexible enough), the choice is entirely yours. Whichever of the exercises you choose, the battle system is very easy to master. And if it's way too easy for you, you can choose to increase the difficulty and intensity –accordingly.

One of the best features in ring fit adventure is the silent mode. The game will ask if you want to be loud or not, and it has other options that you can exchange with, if you are not able to do some specific exercises.

For instance, to go around in the world in Ring Fit Adventure, you have to keep jogging in one position. If you don't want to jog, the game gives you the option of squatting especially if you are a player who does not want to disturb his neighbors. The squatting option is not really any easier, considering the fact that you will have to do like 200-300 squats during your workout session, but it is still worth the while.

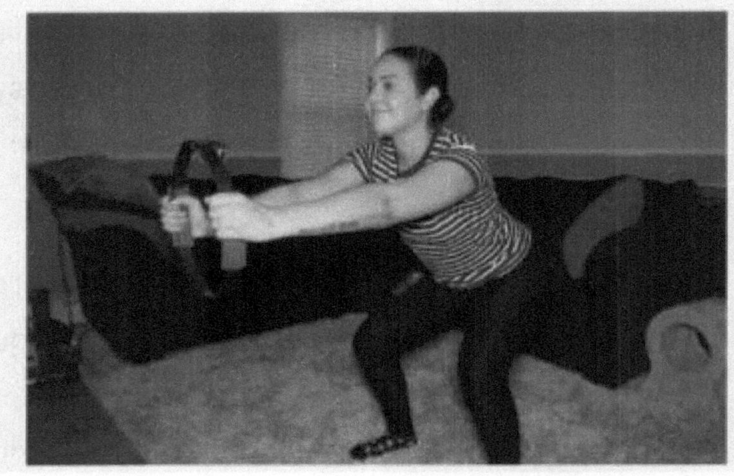

Do not burden yourself with the Ring Fit Adventure game, you will get tired if you allow it. The best I recommend, is to build up in your exercise and watch yourself get better gradually, so that you won't run out of breath.

Take Note that there is a pause button as well- you can always press the button to take a break, ring fit adventure will always ask if you want to take a break after about 15 minutes.

CHAPTER 3: HOW TO SET UP RING FIT ADVENTURE

When you open up the Ring Fit Adventure box, you will find the following items in it: Ring Fit Adventure game, leg strap and Ring Con. To set everything up is pretty simple, just follow the steps below:

1. The ring fit adventure game cartridge should be inserted into your Nintendo switch console
2. Select the ring fit adventure game icon from console Home Menu
   If you have internet connection, you may get prompted to update; you can decide either to do so now or later.
3. Take away the left Joy Con from Nintendo switch system.

4. Slide the left Joy Con into the leg strap pocket with the analog stick at the top and facing outward (as pictured above)

5. On your left thigh, attach the Velcro leg strap to ensure that it is tight enough to stay in place as you move.

6. Once you are ready, stay still and the game will register that your leg strap is in its right place.

7. Take away the right Joy Con from your Nintendo switch system.

8. Hold the Ring Con and look for the protruding black plastic part that has the Nintendo switch logo.

9. Take Note of the "+" symbol on the Joy Con and then slide it into place. It should slide smoothly along the rail and should click into place, just as it does when connecting to the switch console itself.

10.   Put the Ring Con on a flat surface to calibrate it and don't touch it until the game gives you notice that it is okay to do so.

11.   Pick the Ring Con up and squeeze it inward using the two hand grips to proceed. See the picture below.

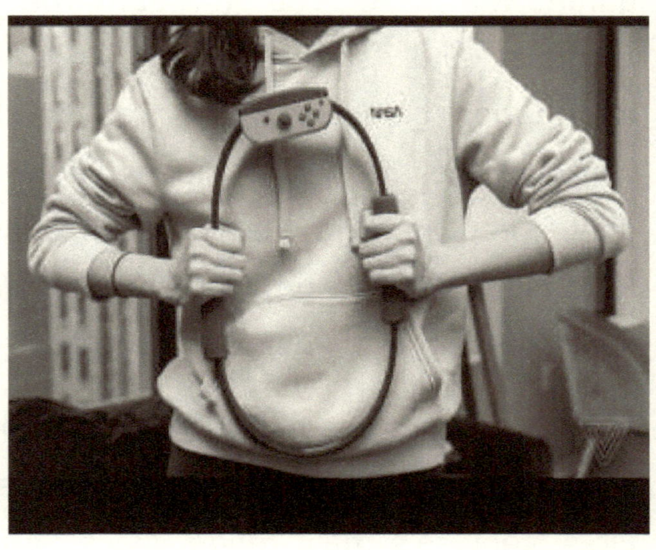

12.   By using the analog stick and buttons on your right Joy Con

(attached to the ring con) select your location.

This will determine how the distance and weight is measured in the game and it can be changed at intervals.

Now that you are at the Ring Fit Adventure main menu, you are ready to begin. The game will take you through the basic controls and some health and safety information before allowing you to choose which of the title's four modes you wish to play. Keep in mind that you can only play Ring Fit Adventure on Nintendo Switch Lite, if you own an extra pair of Joy Cons.

I would recommend that you start out by selecting the Adventure mode which is Ring Fit Adventure's main mode. Once you have selected the mode, you will get a prompting to enter in details on the following: your age, your weight, height and the average level of physical activity that you do.

Make sure you answer truthfully, as this will affect the catered difficulty level you are assigned to and also the estimated calory tracking information. If you are finding the game too easy, you can always adjust the difficulty level (of which there are like 30 of these levels).

The game's adventure mode also introduces the player to an interesting narrative and a list of characters, this is to motivate you further to return for extra workouts in order to see what happens next. When you start the journey, it will just be with a few selected basic exercises, which involves battling with creatures when you are running on the spot to travel through levels, before you will gradually start unlocking more and more levels.

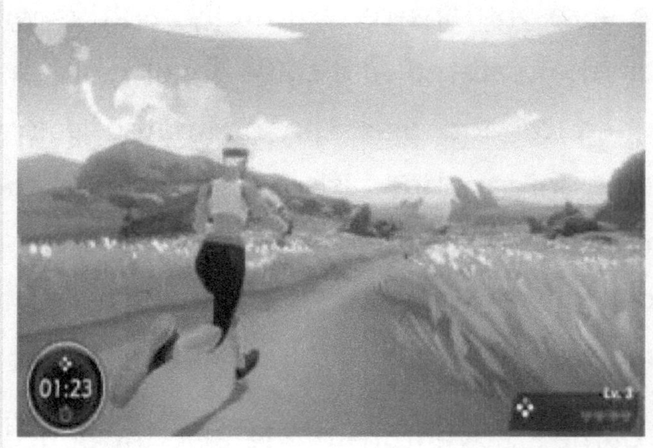

It is possible to focus on workouts which will affect some specific parts of the body, and you can achieve this by customizing your load out.

However, having different varieties of "Fit Skills" equipped will help you get a full body pump on while you are also being prepared for anything.

The color of the enemies you are faced with, represents the type of exercise the different parts of your body will be mostly exposed to.

For example, working with your arms against a red enemy will be more effective whereas you will want to use your legs when facing a blue monster.

CHAPTER 4: GETTING STARTED

But once you actually start playing the game, everything changes. One of the first things you do in Ring Fit Adventure is meeting a sentient ring named... Ring. This Ring functions as both a sidekick and a personal trainer, which will help you through the game with a stable stream of tips and encouragement.

This is how it works: have the leg strap tightened on your leg and hold the Ring-Con in front of you like a steering wheel, then you can move through the level by jogging on the same spot. As you go along, you will constantly meet obstacles that require different movements to overcome them.

If you want to jump, point the Ring Con down and squeeze it; to go up stairs, raise your knees higher while jogging.

Coins can also be collected on the side of the trail by stretching out the Ring Con and sucking them up. Also, you can destroy obstacles such as boxes by squeezing the ring, and this will release a powerful burst of air.

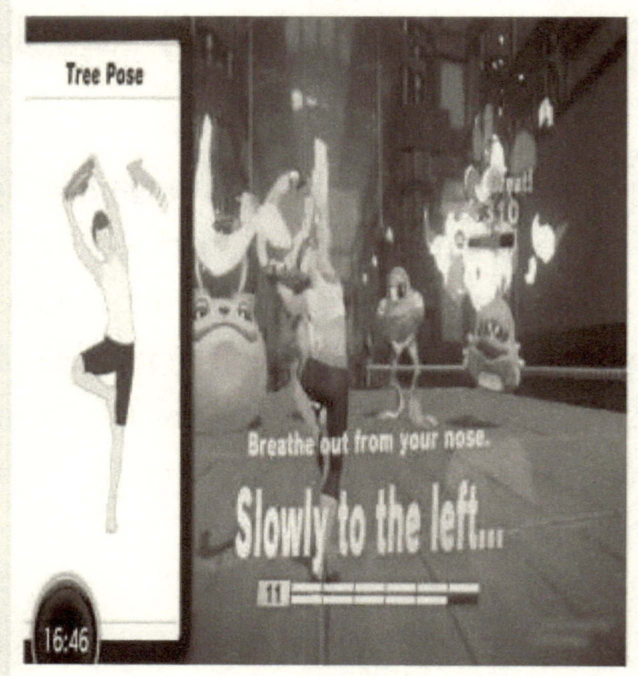

It might sound very easy, but it can also be quite tricky, especially as you will need to remember all of their various inputs all at once, without a pause, from running. Normally, more engagements are added as you make progress.

In the long run, you will be doing squats to jump higher or trampolines and twisting your body in order to paddle a boat. Each level can take from two to 10 minutes, and you may find yourself constantly sweating after doing two or three levels.

Another feature of the game is engaging in battles. Apart from running through each stage, you also have to fight some miscreants. The enemies you fight are a beautiful version of gym gear, like having a trundling kettle-bell with an attitude or a beautiful yoga mat with doe eyes.

The battles are turn-based, looking as if you were playing Final Fantasy in a gym.

For you to be able to attack, you have to select from a range of different exercises. You will then do reps- which could either be squats, a warrior pose, or planking to help you inflict damages on your enemies.

And when it's the turn for your enemies to fight back, you have to hold the ring against your abdomen and squeeze, and you are to hold it for the duration of the attack in order to create a shield. This process will be repeated until one of you run out of strength.

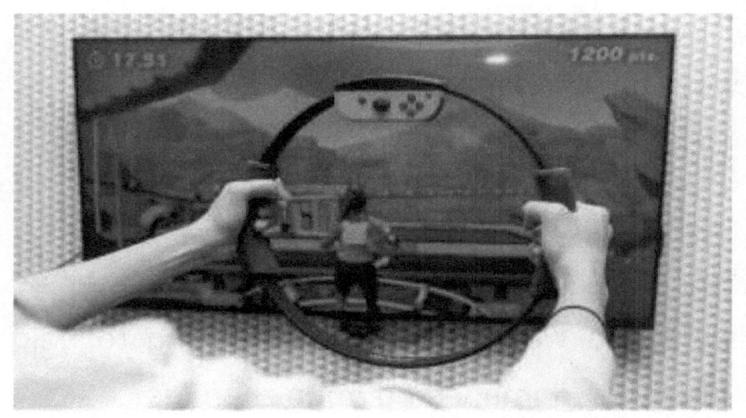

There's a layer of strategy added in to force you to try different exercises. Most enemies have a color, and exercises are also grouped into colors. For example Leg-related exercises are blue, while yoga poses are green. So if you happen to come up against a blue kettle-bell, you may want to do some thigh crunches.

This becomes specifically important against bosses, which have huge health bars. And if you are not being strategic about your attacks, you will definitely have a hard time.

The more you play, the more exercises you will unravel so that you won't get stuck doing the same yoga pose every time you come in contact with an angry green exercise ball.

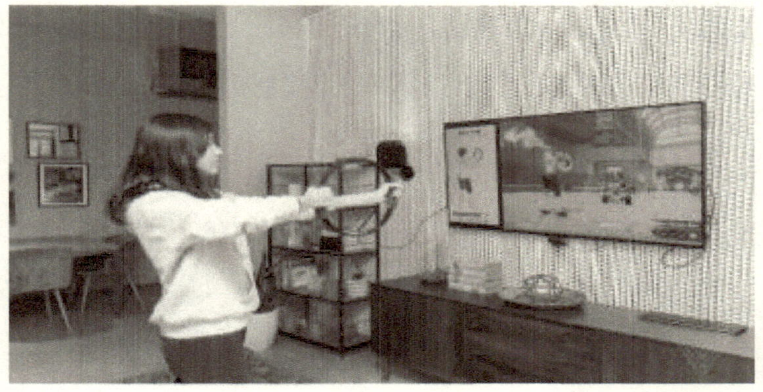

The interesting thing about the game is that, the both halves of Ring Fit Adventure not only work well together, but they feel fully developed on their own. In a unique way, the game will ask you each day if you want to increase the challenge or you want to continue with the normal challenge.

CHAPTER 5: FREQUENTLY ASKED QUESTIONS

CAN I ENGAGE IN THE WORKOUTS OUTSIDE OF THE ADVENTURE MODE

There are different modes in the game. So you can actually do workouts that are outside of the adventure mode. Ring Fit Adventure has a Quick Play mode where you can jump into the exercises of your choice, and where you can also play mini-games, or choose sets of exercises based on the part of your body you want to work on.

WHAT KIND OF WORKOUTS ARE AVAILABLE ON RING FIT

Ring Fit have a lot of different types of exercises across various categories, which are mostly broken down by parts of the body they exercise: chest, legs, arms or yoga poses.

Some of the examples we have seen in trailers so far include squats, bow pulls, overhead lunge twists, thigh presses, hinge poses, chair poses and knee-to-chests. More exercises can be unlocked when you make progress in Adventure mode and leveling up.

CAN I CUSTOMIZE THESE WORK OUTS?

In Ring Fit Adventure, there is some customization that is available that we have seen so far, majorly the kind that allows you to set the level of workout you prefer so that you are not over-working yourself. This mostly comes in the form of a difficulty level selector that goes up in number from 1-30

CAN I PLAY THIS GAME WITH FRIENDS

The peculiarity of the Ring Fit Adventure game is that it is designed as a single-player game and only one player can play per time. Nintendo has encouraged its subscribers in trailers to share the Ring-Con around and play with friends that way but in actual fact there is no true multiplayer.

The game gives you the opportunity to compare scores in various exercises with your friends and with others online to try and obtain the highest score over a period of time.

HOW DOES THE RING CONTROLLER WORK?

The Ring-Con controller is a round exercise ring. It is connected to the Switch when you insert a single Joy-Con into the slot. The other Joy-Con goes into the Leg Strap, which will then detect the motion of your leg, balance and positioning.

The Ring-Con is meant to be squeezed in different ways to do exercises, while the

Joy-Con is to sense the motion and pressure on the Ring-Con to grade your exercises.

IS THE RING CONTROLLER NEEDED TO PLAY THE GAME

You actually need the ring controller to play the game. Ring fit adventure cannot be played without the controller and leg strap, and it is also not sold without the controller or leg strap, so except you are buying the game used, you will always have the controllers to pair with it.

WHAT IS IMPORTANT ABOUT RING FIT ADVENTURE

Ring Fit Adventure is a game that is easy to fit into your life, because each level is just a few minutes long, you can easily do a quick work out on a busy day, but you can also string together a few if you are looking for something tougher.

The game even gives you a warning if it thinks it's time for you to take a break. Ring Fit Adventure also supports multiple accounts, so you can have different people in the same household, using it, and it will track their efforts and customize the experience to their needs. There are also mini-game and customizable exercise playlists for those who don't find it appealing to dig through a multi-hour RPG

CONCLUSION

I can't tell you that Ring Fit Adventure is a proper substitute for going to the gym or a way for you to really get in shape.

What I can say is this: it's a polished, fun game that feels like real workout, and for some persons, it became a way they could almost seamlessly fit in physical activity into their life.

On a final note, it is a good idea to invest in a yoga mat (buy a yoga mat). Some exercises are floor based and incredibly uncomfortable to perform on a hard surface.